Applied Kinesiology Basic 100 Hrs Course

Dr. Andrew Greszczyszyn DC, Phd.

Applied Kinesiology Basic 100 Hrs Course

ISBN 978-1511758314

This work is dedicated to Dr. George Goodheart Jr. Without whom this work could never have been created.

Acknowledgments

Special thanks to my Applied Kinesiology teachers, Dr. Steven Yen my first chiropractic roommate for getting me into interested in Applied Kinesiology and my second room mate Dr. Michael Gorman, who guided much of my advanced learning and ideas which have spurred greater research and advancements of my techniques.

Table of Contents

Course

Applied Kinesiology eCourse

Dr. Andrew Greszczyszyn D.C., PhD.

Dr. Andrew Greszczyszyn DC, Phd.

Applied Kinesiology eCourse

• eCourse Information

• Who I am

• Course

• What Next

• What it is

• AK is a system of using manual muscle test to add to diagnostic value.

• AK does not substitute history, exam, lab work or rational thought, it adds to these!

• Why use AK?

• AK can strengthen diagnostic parameters, and can be a way of treating.

• There are many patterns, therapeutic techniques and tools of healing incorporated in Applied Kinesiology.

• Even one single technique talked about through this course was and can be used as a whole inclusive therapy (from the many disciplines included in AK)

• Imagine a course in Trigger Points, another in Cranial Sacral, another in Chiropractic Adjusting, another in nutrition and allergy testing, maybe another in psychology, one in posture, maybe one in massage, or even one in osteopathy, lymphatic or vasculature drainage.

• It also borrows from Acupuncture Philosophy, Homeopathy, Dentistry, Nutrition, Traditional Chinese Medicine, and even Old School Chiropractic.
  • All these in one system of healing….
  • All this in ONE cCourse!!!

• AK is only as good as the therapist!

- Some people think AK is only as good as the muscle tester....
- THIS IS WRONG!

- Why? Seeing patterns, knowing when to use patters, using techniques talked about in Applied Kinesiology, Listening to the patients history and doing an exam which incorporates patterns
allows one for the most part to speed up practice and even avoid muscle testing during most of the treatment period.

- Some practitioners also use self testing.

- Self testing is using divination or asking questions and receiving guidance not through the patient but through ones own testing on one's self.

- Limitations of this include fear of people finding out you do it, or self imposed limitations that you can not test something or/and your testing parameters which are as great/much as you've learned or test.

- What you know becomes your testing field, unless you ask questions like (other tests, other exams, other treatments, other doctors, other herbs, etc.)

- Dr. George Goodheart Jr. is the Founder of

Applied Kinesiology (AK).

• He was the first chiropractor on a USA Olympic
Team

• He discovered AK, when he noticed a patient of his (delivery man who brought mail to his office) complaining of a winging scapula, and he remembered a muscle test for the serratus anterior muscle (a muscle which holds the scapula to the rib cage).

• Dr. Goodheart tested the serratus anterior muscle on this delivery man and found that it was weak (4/5).

• He then palpated the Origin and Insertion of the weak muscle and noticed that there was painful and nodular bumps.

• He used transverse friction massage and the pain lessened and muscle became strong again!!!

• Dr. Goodheart then began to test all patients
with as many muscle tests as he could

• Using principles like Origin and Insertion, Chapmans' refelexes, Bennettes' reflexes, acupuncture, nutrition, chiropractic, cranial sacral and many other disciplines to treat and make the weak muscles strong again.

• Dr. Goodheart to many and especially to me appears to be an incarnation of healing.

• Just like another icon D.D. Palmer the Founder of Chiropractic (who I will call an incarnation

of healing), Dr. Goodheart noticed patients should be analyzed through examining their structural, chemical and emotional states (similar to D.D Palmers' Trauma, Poison and AutoSuggestion)

• For years Dr. Goodheart used his practice as a way to develop findings in Applied Kinesiology.

• His practice in Michigan became a source of integrating various health practices into a system he later called AK (Applied Kinesiology).

• He helped develop the ICAK (international Council of Applied Kinesiology) released seminars and research tapes, as well as some books on the subject.

• Dr. Goodheart began to get a following and even had an inner circle of teachers he labeled "the dirty dozen"

• This group helped with research, testing and developing the working and seminars which would become the growth of Applied Kinesiology.

• As mentioned AK examines foremost the patient using a Triad of Health.

• Structural, Chemical and Emotional

• Structural Includes: Massage, Orthotics, Nervous and Joints, Cranial Sacral, Lymphatics, Acupuncture, Trigger Points, Muscle Spindles, Vasculature among other things…

• Chemical Includes: allergies, supplements, homeopathy, diet, herbs, nutrition and even things like digestion…

• Emotion Includes: Emotional reflexes and Psychological Reversal to name the most common uses in AK

•   Due to the highly valuable findings and treatment inclusions found in AK many people began to learn and study AK.

•   Some people then took findings and used their own research and methods adopting other techniques….
• Some included NET, TBM, BK, and even others.

•   For the most part they offshooted to remain in either the structural, chemical and emotional side of health, and even now there are more growing subdisciplines in the energetic side of health.

• Who is this Course Designed For?

• The Course is open like AK Courses for anyone that has the ability to Diagnose.

• Given the license to diagnose one could be a psychiatrist, a medical doctor, a chiropractor, and homeopath, a osteopath, a naturopath, a dentist or acupuncturist

• As you can see it is much more than chiropractic.

• Techniques included in AK range from massage, TMJ and Teeth or dentistry, Acupuncture, lymphatic drainage, vascular, cranial sacral, adjusting, trigger point therapy and much more.

• AK and manual muscle testing can help discover other techniques, can help refine techniques, can help decide when to use other techniques and can even provide reason to use a technique(s).

- As AK has grown it has developed a larger following and incorporated more people who have discovered other uses for manual muscle testing.

- What AK really is!
- AK is using manual muscle testing to help strengthen diagnostic criteria in a way to increased the understanding of which, when, how, when and even why to use a therapy.

- Not just a therapy that has been included in AK Basic Course or this course, but any course or therapy you may have learned (with some limitations).

- Finding of recurrent liver problems for example, could suggest to do a blood liver panel, and allergy panel, a detox or even nutrition for the liver.

- As you can see AK is a process of using the mind or intellect and increasing the amount or refinement of diagnosis and then therapy to better aid the patient.

- What AK is not!

- AK is not foo foo, not nonsense, not imaginary and definitely not made up in the mind of the tester.

- True AK practitioners who've been trained and use AK effectively can duplicate and have others with similar instruction duplicate their findings.

- Mastering the techniques is primary to
mastering muscle testing...although mastering
muscle testing is primary to being considered
a good AK or certified AK practitioner.

- Higher than basic training is becoming a Diplomate DIAK (Diplomat International College of Applied Kinesiology).

- One does not need to be a diplomat to be a good practitioner.

- Also one does not have to test each muscle to be a good practitioner

- One does however and should however understand the techniques talked about in
this course (And AK) to become a good healer.

- Secondarily (and often primarily in todays economy) there becomes the need for speed.

- This does not mean short changing a patient...in fact the opposite is true!!!

- Refinement of testing to minimize patient time while giving superior treatment becomes important.

- Seeing patterns, using muscle testing only when needed and refining testing to be used when confounded or looking for a deeper cause.

- This is mastery of Applied Kinesiology.

- Dr. Andrew Greszczyszyn D.C., PhD.

- Doctor of chiropractic, graduated from National University of Health Sciences (formerly National Chiropractic College) in Lombard, Illinois.

- PhD. In Metaphysics

• With over 740 Hrs of Applied Kinesiology Instruction with some of the Top Applied Kinesiologist Doctors

• Teachers include: Dr. Zatkin (worked with Dr. Goodheart), Dr. Bovine, Dr. Tim Francis, Dr. Leaf, Dr. Goodheart, Dr. Schmitt, Dr. Phil Maffetone, Dr. Blaich, NET (Neuroemotional Technique) with Dr. Walker (worked with AK), Acupuncture with Dr. John Amaro (worked with AK)

• Muscle Testing is fundamental to Applied Kinesiology

• Great length could be done to test muscles and learn each muscle

• A muscle test as Dr. Goodheart discovered (as learned in a Book from Dvorak and Dvorak) is a muscle test of any testable muscle by shortening the muscle, testing it against resistance through lengthening or separating its origin/insertion from it's insertion/origin.

• Muscles are then tested individually using a
strong test from any muscle graded as 5/5 and
weak for any muscle testing 4/5 or lower (3/5,
2/5 etc).

• Muscles which do not lock against the testers resistance are then called "weak" muscles.

• One main principle of Applied Kinesiology is that weak muscles (in some cases hypertonic
or super facilitated muscles) cause dysfunction rather than muscles being too "tight"

• What this means is by finding weak muscles or muscles which are graded as 4/5 or lower, one can then determine factors which strengthen those muscles so they become strong again (5/5)

• In short AK was built on each muscle having
five factors which helped strengthen the weak
muscles

• Dr. Goodheart called these the Five Factors of the IVF (intervertebral foramina)

• The five factors include:

• 1) Nerve
• 2) Neurolymphatic
• 3) Neurovasculature
• 4) Cranial Sacral Respiratory   System
• 5) Acupuncture Meridian

• A second main principle in Applied Kinesiology
is that muscles are associated with Organ
Systems.

• This Dr. Goodheart found through the associated Muscle Organ Meridian Association in Chinese Medicine.

• The Following is a Chart to see the Muscle
Organ Associations

- Brain: Supraspinatus
- Eyes/Ears: Upper Trapezius
- Sinus: Neck Flexor/Extensor
- Thymus/Spleen: Middle and Lower Trapezius, Infraspinatus
- Thyroid:Teres Minor
- Parathyroids: Levator Scapulae
- Heart: Subscapularis
- Lungs: Deltoid, Coracoid Bracialis,

- Liver: Pectoralis Sternal Division

- Gallbladder: Popliteus

- Small Intestine: Quadriceps, Adductors

- Large Intestine: TFL, Hamstrings,

- Pancreas: Latissimus dorsi,

- Stomach: Pectoralis Clavicular Division

– Adrenals: Tibialis Posterior, Gastrocnemius,
Soleus,

– Ovaries/Testicles: Gluteus Muscles

– Uterus/Prostate: Gluteus Muscles

– Bladder: Tibialis Anterior, Fibularis Longus/Brevis,

– Kidneys: Psoas,

• Neurolymphatics are generally found
alongside the front of the thorax and along
the posterior spine.

•   A few are located on the head, and also on the pelvis

• The following are locations of common
Neurolymphatics

– Brain: Supraspinatus-External Occipital Protruberance

– Eyes/Ears: Upper Trapezius-Bicepital Groove

– Sinus: Neck Flexor/Extensor-Side of mandible

– Thymus/Spleen: Middle and Lower Trapezius, Infraspinatus-Right of xyphoid in intercostal space

– Thyroid:Teres Minor-1st intercostal space

– Parathyroids: In body of Teres Muscles/lateral border scapulae

– Lymphatics: Pec. Minor-Sternum and Xyphoid

– Heart: Subscapularis-2nd intercostal space

– Lungs: Deltoid, Coracoid Bracialis, -Coracoid process

– Liver: Pectoralis Sternal Division-8th intercostal space, on right/below nipple

– Gallbladder: Popliteus-Intercostal (1 and 2) below

Liver Neurolymphatic (9-10th intercostal space right)

– Small Intestine: Quadriceps, Adductors-left and right lower ribs

– Large Intestine: TFL, Hamstrings,-Tensor Fascia Latae and T12 rib ends left right

– Pancreas: Latissimus dorsi, -Left 9/10th intercostal space

– Stomach: Pectoralis Clavicular Division-left 8th intercostal space

– Adrenals: Tibialis Posterior, Gastrocnemius, Soleus,-1 inch out 2 inches up from umbilicus (right and left respective)

– Ovaries/Testicles: Gluteus Muscles-pubic symphysis right left

– Uterus/Prostate: Gluteus Muscles-pubic symphysis right left

– Bladder: Tibialis Anterior, Fibularis Longus/Brevis,- pubic symphysis centre
– Kidneys: Psoas,-T11 rib ends right left

• Neurovasculature points are treated when
they are positive (touching them makes a
weak muscles test strong)

• They are treated by rubbing them in a circulature fashion for 30-45 seconds

• As they become treated they will become less painful, less nodular, and more relaxed.

• Neurovasculature points are generally found on the head.
• The following are locations of common
Neurovasculatures
• Diaphragm-bregma and lamdoidal

- Stomach/Emotion- 2 inches above eye pupils center righ/left

- Others using Walter AK Synopsis or AK wall chart from Systems DC (ICAK website)

- Neurovasculature points are treated when they are positive (touching them makes a weak muscles test strong)

- They are treated by holding them using a light pressure until a pulse is felt, generally 30-45 seconds up to a couple minutes.

- The pulse felt under the fingers is indication they have been treated...along side a non responsive muscle test (meaning the weak muscle remains weak with touching this point, or the muscle is now strong and touching the point keeps it strong)

- What is a Cranial Fault?

- A cranial Fault is a abnormal motioning skull bone, or a skull bone which is fixed and non moveable.
- Remember the skull is not one bone.

- Also remember that the skull moves through various ranges of motion as the cerebrospinal fluid is moved through the ventricles of the skull and through the spinal column, as the patient/person breathes normally.

- Is a bone in the skull is fixed or does not move correctly it will cause a muscle testing change as the patient alters the phases of respiration

- For instance with a inspiratory assist cranial fault a weak muscle will test strong after the patient inhales and holds their breath during the test.

- The following are the indications for testing cranial faults

- Inspiration assist: a weak muscles tests strong after the patient inhales and holds their breath
- Expiration assist: a weak muscles tests strong after the patient exhales and holds the breath out

- Pituitary Drive Inspiration: a weak muscle tests strong after a patient maximally inspires and holds a forced inspiration in

- Pituitary Drive Expirations: a weak muscles tests strong after a patient maximally expires and holds a forced expiration out

• Temporal Bulge: a weak muscles tests strong
after the patient exhales fully and holds a half
breath in

• Parietal Descent: a weak muscles tests strong after the patient
inhales fully and lets out a half breath

• Nasophenoid: a weak muscles tests strong
after the doctor challenges or presses the
corner of the bridge of the nose (one direction
at a time, either left to right, or right to left).

• Frontal: a weak muscles tests strong after the patient pulls down
on the front (immediate front, left or right (one at a time) top tooth)-
upper central.

• Inspiratory Assist: On inspiration move the occiput from
posterior to anterior on the side of weakness.

• Expiratory Assist: On expiration move the occiput from anterior
to posterior on the side of weakness.

- Pituitary Drive: Before correction determine which of either the or a) the thyroid Neurolymphatic b) the adrenal gland Neurolymphatic OR c) the sexual reproductive glands Neurolymphatic cause a muscle to be weak, and are strengthened (still contact that point) while simultaneously contacting the bregma or Third Eye which is the Pituitary Point.

- Once you know if it is thyroid, adrenal, or sex hormones that are the problem, perform the corrective phase of respiration and cranial correction (inspiratatory: mastoid P-A, expiratory: mastoid A-P) while the patient holds both pituitary and affective hormone (that was problem) which was either the thyroid, adrenal, sex hormones

- Do the breathing for 3-5 minutes, using forced breathes. About every 30seconds stop and rub the pituitary point like a NeuroLymphatic

- Temporal Bulge: Apply a A-P and P-A force on the skull on the side of weakness (normally the left side of the skull-the side is often apparent by a temporal bulge or banana head), while the patient takes a breath out, maximizing the force towards the center of the convexity as the patient reaches half exhalation.

- Parietal Descent: Apply a inferior to superior force on the side of lession/weakness (normally the right side of the skull-the side which is concave), while the patient takes a breath in, maximizing the force towards the top of the head as the patient reaches half inhalation.

- Notice do not jam the sagittal suture at the top of the head, instead block the skull from jamming using the opposite hand (this normally means applying a force to prevent the right temporal bone from jamming into the suture from the right side).

- Nasopheniod: On the phase of breath that corrected a right or left nasophenoid challenge, press the nasophenoid that direction on the corrective phase of respiration.

- Frontal: On the side of weakness 1st: pull down the inside central top gumline on side of weakness 2nd, pull down laterally the top molar gumline/at the pterygoid pocket on the side of weakness (being careful not to fracture the
hamate bone) 3rd: push up/superior the pterygoid on the side opposite weakness

- What is a Sacral Fault?

- A sacral Fault is a abnormal motioning sacral bone, or a sacral bone which is fixed and non moveable.

- Remember the sacrum is a bone which allows movement greater than nutation and counternutation.

- Also remember that like the skull bones which move through various ranges of motion, the sacral bone moves and helps propel cerebrospinal fluid back up the spine to the brain and ventricles of the skull as the patient/person breathes normally.

- Inspiration assist: a weak muscles tests strong after the patient inhales and holds their breath OR the sacral bone on the right/left (one at a
   time) is challenged/moved into a counternutation direction.
- Expiration assist: a weak muscles tests strong
   after the patient exhales and holds the breath out
   OR the sacral bone on the right/left (one at a
   time) is challenged/moved into a nutation
   direction.

• Inspiratory: on the side of weakness during
inspiration, move the sacrum into
counternutation.

• Expiratory: on the side of weakness during expiration, move the
sacrum into nutation (a hand at apex, and hand at base of sacrum on
given side)

• Dural Torque: C1-4 (either on the right or left
TP's) are pulled superior as the coccyx is
moved inferior, causing a muscle to test weak.

• Indications: sore, palpatory C/s C1-4 on right or left, too much
protein, tight muscles, inflexibility, cranial faults, TMJ, and even Pelvic
Categories.

• Treatment: Raise or move the coccyx superior
towards the C/spine at an angle that
decreases the palpatory (right or left sided C1-
C4 TP pain), as you raise the coccyx superior,
move the C1-4 SP inferior towards the coccyx.

• Then I adjust subluxations at L3, T10, T5/6 and upper C/s

Switching/Neurological
Disorganization

• What is Neurological Disorganization?

• Often called switching, it is a disorganization of the left and right hemispheres of the brain, not working in synch.

Switching

• It is more that a mix up of left and rights, although this is often indicated when it is present.

• Switching can cause memory problems, learning problems, the sense of struggling for energy, mixing things up, drained energy, limitations of strength, limitations of health, mixing left and right up, dyslexia, ADD, ADHD, autism, among other hormonal abnormalities, and muscles imbalances!

Testing Switching

• Switching is generally tested using a two hand Bilateral K27 (Kidney Acupuncture Point 27) which is at the sternoclavicular border on the right side and left side simulataneously.

• If contact at these two points (together) cause a weakness in muscle strengthen then switching or neurological disorganization is indicated.

Original Treatment of Neurological
Disorganization

• The original treatment was to rub the K27 points simultaneously like a NeuroLymphatic.

• Other techniques have been introduced.

• The following two will be described in this course.

• 1) Dr. Francis' Ocular Lock

• 2) Dr. Schmitt's IRT (Injury Recall Technique)

Ocular Lock

- Dr. Tim Francis an AK diplomat teaches that ocular lock is present in most if not all cases of switching.

- It is a good idea to treat every patient for ocular lock as the first step in treatment.

• The following is the patterns for ocular lock.

 – Eyes UP
 – Eyes DOWN
 – Eyes UP LEFT
 – Eyes UP RIGHT
 – Eyes DOWN LEFT
 – Eyes DOWN RIGHT

– Eyes LEFT

– Eyes RIGHT

– ONE eye CLOSED

– OTHER eye CLOSED

– TONGUE out

– Eyes UP: Atlanto-Occiput Flexion, Nutation

– Eyes DOWN: B/L inferior Occiput (correction), Counternutation

– Eyes UP LEFT: Occiput Left
– Eyes UP RIGHT: Occiput Right
– Eyes DOWN LEFT: Sacrum Left
– Eyes DOWN RIGHT: Sacrum Right

– Eyes LEFT: C2 Left

– Eyes RIGHT: C2 Right

– ONE eye CLOSED: Atlas

– OTHER eye CLOSED: Atlas

– TONGUE out: Hyoid (then challenge or palpate), Correction

• Corrects Top, down, Inside, Out!

• Atlanto/Occiput, Nutation, back up B/L inf.
Occiput. Counternation, back up occiput,
sacrum, up C2 down…then energetics at C1
and Hyoid (inside out)!!!

• Often times scars or injuries cause switching
to reoccur.

• Dr. Wally Schmitt teaches IRT (injury recall technique) as a way
to overcome neurological disorganization!

• Dr. Schmitt challenges the K27 points with B/L
hand contacts of various varieties.

• 1) K27

• 2) K27 with hands crossed, but arms and forearms not touching

- 3) K27 with Knuckles of fingers

- 4) K27 with Knuckles of fingers crossed, but arms and forearms not touching

- 2) K27 with hands crossed, but arms and forearms not touching: Scar or injury (like Burn or Fracture) somewhere on the body

- 3) K27 with Knuckles of fingers: Cranial Faults

- 4) K27 with Knuckles of fingers crossed, but arms and forearms not touching: Teeth/Wisdom Teeth Scars

- Treating the injury or the scar using IRT is the treatment.

- Touch, rub, palpate, or stimulate the scar, or area of injury and then "flick" the talus on the side of lesion, moving the talus in an inferior direction-decompressing the ankle mortise joint. For axial or skull IRT flex the atlanto- occipital joint (instead of the ankle mortise joint).

- The following are some of the causes of Switching which cause Switching/Neurological Disorganization to happen or reoccur.
  - 1) Allergies
  - 2) Chemicals
  - 3) Additives
  - 4) Injuries
  - 5) Scars
  - 6) Herbs
  - 7) Drugs

- Notice: It is important to correct neurological disorganization, and also important to find higher correction (Ocular Lock/IRT) however it is even more important to find the Primary Cause(s) of the cause of the Switching Problem
  - 1) Allergies
  - 2) Chemicals
  - 3) Additives
  - 4) Injuries
  - 5) Scars
  - 6) Herbs
  - 7) Drugs

• There are two main principle of chemistry.

• 1: Too Much of Something

• 2: Not Enough of Something

• The Something could be a nutrient, a chemical, a vitamin, water, fat, carbohydrate, protein, toxin, etc.

• Nutrients can be tested to determine if they are needed by the body.

• If a weak muscle tests strong after testing a nutrient, it is indicated that the nutrient is something the body is needing.

• Confirmation is using a Temporal Tap (on the left side) which is tracing the Temporal Sphenoid Line (see accompanying diagram next slide), in a clockwise direction (with patient facing the anterior direction), which maintains a strong muscle test after tasting or smelling the nutrient or tested vitamin, mineral, water, homeopathy, etc.

Temporal Sphenoid Line (Actually the
insertions of the temporalis muscle)

Testing Toxins

- Similarly is a toxin is added to the tongue, skin, or nose/smell and this chemical causes a strong muscle to test weak we can say it is toxic to the body/individual.

Nutrients

- The following is a short list of common muscle/organ associated nutrients

– Brain: Supraspinatus-DNA/RNA

– Eyes/Ears: Upper Trapezius-Vitamin A

– Thymus/Spleen: Middle and Lower Trapezius, Infraspinatus-Zinc, Vitamin A,

– Thyroid:Teres Minor-iodine, EFA's

– Parathyroids: Lev. Scapulae-Calcium

– Lymphatics: Pec. Minor-zinc, water

– Heart: Subscapularis-Hawtorn, CoQenzyme, Carnitine

– Lungs: Deltoid, Coracoid Bracialis, -Vitamin C

– Liver: Pectoralis Sternal Division-B Complex

– Gallbladder: Popliteus-Vitamin B, Beta Carotene

– Small Intestine: Quadriceps, Adductors-Vitamin D

– Large Intestine: TFL, Hamstrings,-glutamine, Vitamin E

– Pancreas: Latissimus dorsi, -chromium, pancreatic enzymes

– Stomach: Pectoralis Clavicular Division-digestive enzymes, Betaine HCl

– Adrenals: Tibialis Posterior, Gastrocnemius, Soleus,-B5, B6, Licorice, Vitamin C, Choline

– Ovaries/Testicles: Gluteus Muscles-glandulars tissue

– Uterus/Prostate: Gluteus Muscles-saw palmetto

– Bladder: Tibialis Anterior, Fibularis Longus/Brevis,- Vitamin A

– Kidneys: Psoas,-water

• The third part of Triad of Health is Emotions

• Original AK could be considered "weak" in this area of treatment but is still functional

• Traditionally it uses the Stomach Neurovascular Points to treat emotional problems.

• To test and see if the emotions are problematic get the patient to cover their forehead with a hand and see if it makes a strong muscle go weak

• If it does it is indicated to treat the problematic emotion using the stomach neurovasculature as the patient thinks about the emotional limitation.

• Once the pulse is felt below each set of fingers then the emotion is not problematic (ie. The patient can think about the emotion but will not become "stressed" about it, or may not even think about it again)

• AK is good as it does not need to talk about the emotional limitation, getting the patient to Think of the situation that is bothering them.

• AK is bad because unless the patient knows what is bothering them emotionally then it could take extra time to test each emotion to get the right one/needed correction.

• Two other offshoot techniques are great to fit in and correct Emotional Limitations

• 1) NET (NeuroEmotional Technique-Dr. Scott Walker)-generally for limiting beliefs

• 2) PsychoKinesiology-generally for desires (see Kindle eCourse by Dr. Andrew Greszczyszyn for this information)

• A good way to see if there are feet subluxation is to tap (like the anvil orthopedic test) the bottom of the foot and test a previously strong muscle to see if it goes weak.

• If it goes weak after tapping the bottom of the foot, that foot could generally be said to have feet subluxations.

• Palpate or challenge the foot bones to see if there are subluxations. Adjust and correct, then test to make sure the anvil test does not weaken a previously strong muscle.

• During normal walking gait as the left (right) arm move forward the right leg (left) comes forward as well. As this happens, the right (left) arm moves back and the left leg (right) is in the back position.

• This means:

• 1. with right leg forward...left lat should test weak.

• 2. with left leg forward...right lat should test weak.

• 3. with right leg forward...left pec clavicular should test weak

• 4. with left leg forward...right pec clavicular should test weak

• If these patterns of normal gait do not test correctly, examine illiolumbar ligament on side of lesion and correct with Origin Insertion, or Muscle Spindle Activity.

• Illeocecal Valve is an important consideration in AK.

• It is a part of the digestive system between the small intestine and large intestine.

• This functional valve should allow food stuff to move from small intestine to large intestine BUT not back
• Often times is gets stuck open or stuck closed
(open valve, closed valve)

• Test a previously strong muscle to see if goes
week by manually opening the valve (right sided
lower right quadrant abdomen) pushing in and
down to the outside or side (right)…to close it
challenge in and up to the left shoulder…

• There is a valve of Huston which acts similar to the ICV (although is found on the left side of the abdomen…between the large bowel and rectum).

• The following are some indications: allergies,
dark circles under the eyes, lethargic,
switching, pain in unusual places, morning
pain or morning fatigue, weight gain,
bloatiness, foot sweating and smell,
headaches, and general body odor

- Examine and treat the NL for valve which are poster right sided C3-5 TP, Inguinal fossa anterior right thigh, Kidney 3 and Bladder 57 acu points, Anterior L1 and C5 subluxations, NL over valve huston and ICV...emotions dogmatic position

- Nutrition examine and avoid allergies, support bowel health with glutamine and vitamin D, Vitamin C

• Rub NL Small Intestine, C3/L3 subluxation, NL over Valves

- Using wrist pulse points with thumb thenar as GV/CV, left side upper as Small Intestine (Heart), slightly below that Gallbaldder (Liver), an little more below that Bladder (Kidney)

- Right side it is thenar CV/GV, below that on wrist crease Large Intestine (Lung), slightly below that Stomach (Spleen) and a little below that Triple Warm (Circulation Sex)
  • NOTE: (in parenthesis are deeper pressure)

• Examine which pulse point (left side or right side and each position) causes a strong muscle to become weak or a weak muscle to become strong…this is the acupuncture meridian that needs balancing.

• Next test the Associated Alarm point to confirm…and a weak organ associated muscle to see if they are weak.

• If the associated muscle and alarm point test positive then examine tonification or sedation point as negating the weak muscle or alarm point test…treat the positive one (makes a weak muscle go strong) using rubbing, pressing, moxibustion, needling, electricity, laser, etc.

• Also adjust joint in close proximity to acupuncture point, alarm point and associated point on Governing Vessel (Spine and Associated Vertebrae Adjusting)

• If there is recurrent or multiple points on pulse diagnosis treat C0, C1, C2 first (also switching) and examine and balance diaphragm, plus hydration.

• In AK there are three pelvic categories (Cat I, Cat II, Cat III)

• Sacral Boot Fixation

• Examine this using two hand therapy localization (touching with both hands over the right or left SI joint).

• If this touch of both hands over the SI joint (either left or right joint) causes a muscle to test weak it suggest CAT I

• With a CAT I, then press the left PSIS and right Ishium OR right PSIS and left Ishium and test for weakening of a muscle...the one that weakness the muscle is the one that needs to be treated...

• Next block using Dejarnnete blocks under the right anterior lower thigh and anterior left upper thigh when there was weakening of pressing a challenge on right PSIS and left ishium (remember patient is prone for CAT I testing) OR... left anterior lower thigh and anterior right upper thigh in left PSIS and right Ishium challenge weakness. (NOTE challenge by moving the PSIS and Ishium on opposite sides Posterior to Anterior in a bouncing motion-then test the opposite PSIS Ishim combination) NOTE not same side but opposite PSIS and Ishium challenge.

- Let the patient rest on these blocks and pump the Side opposite the lesion (SIDE OF POSITIVE CAT I) not over a block

- Do it until a simultaneous bilateral hamstring tests weak together...then unblock the patient sliding out both blocks at the same time. (NOTE SAME TIME).

- Also check for lateral atlas, which is common to this fixation.

- A category two upper SI subluxation or Posterior Ilium has finding of medial knee pain (PES ansinus, gacilis and Sartorius insertion)...upper inguinal fossa pain and short leg length (NOTE Unless they are switched...these three finding should be present if not unswitch patient first).

- In lower SI subluxation Anterior Superior Ilium the finding is long leg length, lateral knee pain and lower inguinal fossa pain.

• Note you can do a muscle test and one hand touching the SI joint (upper and lower) to see if it is present then check for the triad of leg length, fossa pain and knee side pain.

• Treating a CAT II can be done side laying using drops, kick pulls, or even blocks...

• If the patient has recurrent problems of SI joints or the finding of pain in fossa, leg length and knee side pain don't resolve Treat a CAT III first.

• CAT III is a lumbopelvis subluxation.

• To test it challenge the L5 SP left to right as you pull posterior on the anterior thigh on the side you are moving the SP towards...

• SP moving left to right, pull A-P on right side of anterior thigh.

• SP moving right to left, pull A-P on left side of anterior thigh.

• Then test a muscle. If it goes weak then CAT III is present.

• To treat the CAT III (still prone) block using Dejarnette blocks under the anterior superior iliac spine facing or angled in direction that you moved SP (on left side in left to right SP challenge weakness...right side in right to left SP challenge weakness) and the second block under the anterior lower thigh on the opposite side of the first block (angled towards the tip of the first block).continued...

• The slowly adjust the second block (right side in left position 1st block...left side in right position 1st block) to become parallel to the first block...monitoring Piriformis pain and slowly adjusting this block as pain diminishes.

• To test and see if the lumbar facets are imbricated (overlapping one another) you test a muscle on side of suspicious imbrication and push a straight leg into the lumbar spine

(moving the leg away from the body but in
same line as body helps jam the lumbar facet
together)…if this causes a weakness there is a
facet on that side of challenge.

- Block the lumbar perpendicular to the body under the facet of
Lumbar and yank the leg on side of imbrication caudally (toward the end
of the table).
  - This will separate the facets

- Then do a rolfing or flushing massage (stripping) to the
quadratus lumborum on side of Imbrication.

- Then do transverse frictional massage to Origin and Insertion of
Quadratus muscle on imbrication side (lower ribs and iliac crest).

- There are subluxations…which is one joint or
one vertebrae that is maligned, malposition or
subluxed.

- This is not a fixation.

• A fixation is a group (at least two adjacent and or both upper and lowe iliac (SI joints on one side) that are fixed as a group and move as a group yet are fixed together.

• There can be fixation at CO-C/s, Upper C/s. Lower C/s, C/T, T/s, L/s, Iliac

• Most often there are bilateral muscle weakness patterns that lead you to find fixations

• This is slow…Instead use motion palpation and move SP left to right above and below a subluxation (or restricted vertebrae) to see if the pattern is there….the following is the patterns

• Move an SP left to right and then right to left.

• The direction it will not move (if it is fixed) is labeled as posterior side (won't move toward posterior side).

• Next motion the TP's on left side and right side.

• The side it won't move into (won't move P-A on) is the side you name.

• Left to right fixed…P-A fixed on left…called a
left anterior

• Left to right fixed…P-A fixed on right…called a right posterior

• Right to left fixed…P-A fixed on left…called a left posterior

• Right to left fixed…P-A fixed on right…called a right posterior

• Adjust a fixation using B/L (two hand crossed hand contacts)…

• In Posterior fixations adjust the upper most fixed veterbrae on the one below it (contact the upper posterior side and the one below it's anterior side)

• In Anterior fixation adjust the lower most fixed veterbrae on the one above it (contact the lower posterior side and the one above it's anterior side).

• Adjust these using a Mennel's side laying adjustment. (Check the eCourse on Adjusting on soon to be added on Agreszcz/youtube channel).

• In diaphragm test a muscle after getting the patient to suddenly stop their breath (not hold a breath in or out) while they touch the xiphoid.

• If this causes a muscle weakness adjust T/L fixation and use the lambdoid and bregma Neurovasculars, as well as adjust C3-5 subluxations (phrenic) and T10 (Merrick level)

• To test if there is a hiatal hernia problem (often seen in heart burn, digestive problems or bloatiness and gas) move the diaphragm (palpate under the xyphoid on the left side under the rib cage) in and upwards…

• If this motion causes a strong muscle to test weak, then it is positive for Hiatal Hernia.

• To treat it, press in again as the patient exhales, then maintain this position and allow them to breath in then push deeper on expiration (do this repetition three or four times) maintaining the deep attained on expiration and going deep posterior on expiration…

• Then on the last exhalation tug caudally (towards the feet)…

• This can be done standing for action of gravity.

• One can test this through muscle testing the pec minor muscle (see eCourse on Muscle testing) and getting the patient to raise the legs and pelvis while supine forcing lymph to back up in the head.

• If this position causes the pec minor muscle to test weak (from a previously strong pec minor without the retrograde position) then it is positive for retrograde lymphatic treatment

• You can also test pec minor in the clear if weak there likely is a lymphatic problem…

• If the pec minor muscles are not weak...then test them after stretching the pec minor muscle...if this tests weak do Origin and Insertion of Pec minor muscle, fascial flush (rolfing or stripping the pec minor) and rub Neurolymphatics along the Sternum, Manubrium and Xyphoid.

• Tell the patient to drink more water, and test for the need of zinc

Retrograde or Lymphatics Indications

• If there is many neurolympatics the patient either needs more water or retrograde treatment done (likely both need treatment).

• This is the case of older patients, patients that work out chest (push ups, bench press or have tight chest muscles), people that don't drink water and those that are deficient in zinc.

Lovett Brothers

- There is a concept of the subluxation complex where the spine becomes subluxed in a pattern.

• The pattern occurs sometimes as follows

• C1/L5   C2/L4 C3/L3 C4/L2
• C5/L1   C6/T12   C7/T11   T1/T10
• T2/T9   T3/T8 T4/T7 T5/T6
• CO/Sacrum   Sphenoid/Coccyx

Importance of Lovett

• If there is a recurrent subluxation, examine it's Lovett partner.

• It often is subluxed

• For those unable or do not wish (hopefully just the case of patients) to adjust Coccyx then balance the sphenoid this often is enough

- Ribs and Metatarsals may have a correlation similar to Lovett

TMJ

• To test TMJ, Touch the TMJ joint with three finger (not thumb) and test a strong muscle to see if it goes weak (or goes weak after the patient bites down, opens wide, moves jaw forward, to either side (test both) or retracts the jaw).
   • Opening weakness is internal ptyergoid problem
   • Closing is master or temporalis

• Sides of these muscle can be appreciated by which side you are moving the jaw toward, opening or closing while touch a side (use anatomy).

TMJ treatment

• Generally use Origin Insertion (transvers massage) and/or facial flush (rolfing, stripping)

• There are two types (Dr. Goodheart was working on the third type before his passing on)

• Strain Counter Strain

• Fascial Flush

• This is a trigger point in a muscle that is present when a strong muscle test weak after the muscle is contracted then tested again.

• The way to treat it is us positional release by putting pressure over the Trigger Point which shortening the muscle...one needs to know anatomy of the muscle and identify which muscle the Trigger point is in...then test the muscle, contract the muscle, then test the muscle again.

• Treatment is shortening the muscle while putting pressure over the Trigger Point and holding for 30-45 seconds in the shortened position.

• This is a trigger point in a muscle that is present when a strong muscle test weak after the muscle is stretched then tested again.

• The way to treat it is use fascial flush, rolfing or stripping the muscles over the Trigger Point or body of the muscle. One needs to know anatomy of the muscle and identify which muscle the Trigger point is in…then test the muscle, stretch the muscle, then test the muscle again.

• Treatment again is stripping the muscle.

• Strain counter strain may require Folic Acid

• Fascial Flush may require B12.

• Occasionally the teeth become subluxed.
• Touch a tooth and test to see if it causes weakness.
Touching at the gumline is best.
• If it test weak, then move that tooth in a direction until you find weakness…this is the direction you use for correction.

• Next find the phase (inspiration or expiration) that negates the directional weakness (strengthens that weakness causes by the direction the tooth was moved in)

- Next push the tooth in the needed direction only on the phase of respiration that negated the muscle weakness

- Test quadriceps muscles with eyes open and then eyes closed.

- If the quads test weak after closing the eyes, this is need to treat pineal glands.

- Rub Small Intestine Neurolymphatics (lower rib border) with eyes closed.

- May need to test nutrition for pineal (building blocks) or take melatonin (remember this is not long term as it is a hormone).

- Headaches at top of head.
- Test to see if the prostate or uterine is dropped…supine press in an slightly above the pubic symphysis, moving
  it caudally (towards feet)…then test a strong muscle
- If it goes weak you should treat this.
- On expiration push in and up (slightly above the pubic symphysis) as the patient raised arms above head, and legs off table into flexion (hips)
- Then the patient relaxes as inspires (back to table)
  while doctor does not press into the lower abdomen.
- Repeat a few times.

• STANDING P-A

• High shoulder: think weak lattisimus

• High Hip: think weak sartoris, quads, gracilis

• High shoulder, hip and occiput same side:
think weak glut med same side

• High occiput, contralateral high should, High
Hip (same side occiput): think CAT III

• SUPINE

• Leg Turned Out-Think Weak TFL

•   Bilateral Weak TFL-think Iron deficiency anemia

•   Leg Turned in…Think Weak Psoa muscle same side (occiput)

• Accompanying Muscle Testing Videos will be added shortly to agreszcz (youtube channel)

• To be added to the AK mailing list of information, new patterns, research and additions to this course email agreszcz@Hotmail.com with Applied Kinesiology Information in the subject line.